How to survive working in Home Health Nursing

By: Olivia Layne

Table Of Contents

1. Introduction
2. Pros of working home health
3. Different types of home health cases
4. The CPS Nurse
5. The at home full time parent cases
6. The working parents cases
7. G - Tube Cases
8. Trach patient cases
9. Some Advice

How to Survive Home Health Nursing

This is a short and sweet ebook on how to survive Home Health Care. As you do know there is a shortage of nurses and there are valid reasons to why there is. I will break it down so you get an idea on why and what is currently going on in the nursing world. Brace yourself because it gets real. The truth of working home health. The pros and the cons along with some real examples from nurses that lived through it. Remember someone always has a story to tell. Listen to them and take notes so you can be prepared for it all.

If you are a nurse that means you worked hard to get that degree/license. You would do whatever it takes to protect it. I honestly don't blame you one bit. Unfortunately there are people out there in the world that want to see you fail for no reason at all. Only because they are jealous or not capable of achieving it themselves. Not realizing that you put in all the hard work and dedication to obtain that degree. You must realize that there will always be people around that love what you do and some that hate you just because. That's why they say "You must have thick skin".

With this ebook I will teach you how to do your part and not let the negative people get you down nor hinder your success in the workplace. You will know your true potential and how it will help you in your journey to success. Never underestimate yourself or your abilities to overcome the hurdles that life has. You are a winner, believer, mother, father, son, daughter. You're an all around wonderful person. If you believe it you will feel it and that's when you start to bloom and flourish.

Now make sure you always remember that everyone experiences different things along the way. Some of us have similar stories to tell, while others experience things differently. If you made it this far you love doing what you do obviously. If you're just starting out or on your journey to become a nurse, do know it is worth it. It will be difficult but anything too easy is not worth it at all. You will put in blood, sweat and tears along the way and when you're a nurse. Never give up and never give in. You will make it. If you get knocked down, get back up and try a different approach to things. Never stick to the same way of doing things. Especially knowing it didn't work the first time you tried it that way. Welcome to the nursing side of the world ladies and gents.

Now let's make it clear, nursing is not easy no matter where you work. A little about my background as a nurse. I worked overnight at an Assisted Living facility and that was a nightmare. It was a nightmare because you will always have to deal with lazy people not wanting to do their job. I was the head nurse of 4 CNA's and each floor had a CNA. Each floor had twenty something people. The CNA's were on point at times but there was always one that would do what she wanted to do and didn't care. When I had a discussion with the head nurse on how we should handle the situation she agreed. Basically the CNA would go to sleep in the recliner meant for the patients and every time I came to do my rounds she was asleep. I reported it to the head nurse. They had a discussion with her and she was given another chance but they did say this was a problem they've been having for a while now.

So I go into work believing things would change, NOPE. I did my rounds and there she was fast asleep. When I continued to check my patients and do what was needed a patient was on the floor. He had fallen while trying to get out of his bed. I immediately assisted the patient, assessed and had to make a report. Patient was okay, thank goodness but the CNA should have been awake to assist this patient with his needs. I made sure to let the head nurse know of the incident via report in the morning. She was upset and she made it clear that the CNA days were numbered.

When I was collecting my things to go home another nurse came to me and wanted to talk. This nurse was in her late 60's early 70's. She basically said we need that CNA here. She accepts shifts when no one else does. We are already short staff and if she is gone we will be really short staff. This seasoned nurse was really upset with me. I had to say my peace in a professional way. I think she was stunned when I asked her " So you're telling me it's more important to have a body here but not quality work to secure the safety of the patients in this facility'? If you could have seen the look on her face. Priceless. She said " Oh no, uumm wait. It doesn't sound good but we need her. So from that point on I knew it would be a problem and I refused to continue to work for that company. I explained that I worked hard for my license and will not put it into jeopardy for such carelessness and ignorance. They tried to get me to come back but I refused and moved on.

I honestly felt like "What is this world coming to"? How can you choose just having a body there and not the welfare of the actual patients? I worked with Travel Hospice and a Travel nurse in my city. I really enjoyed it and it's something you can do if you don't mind driving. Some areas on your list you are sent to are questionable but I made it to and from with no issues. Someone explained to me to try Home Health and I really was not interested at all. I loved what I was doing and it paid me well. But somehow my friend, who is a nurse herself convinced me to give it a try.

Let's just say I really was not ready for what would be the start of a crazy nursing life of home health. Now I learned early on to never just work with one Home Health Agency. You should work with at least two to three. I know that might be crazy but let me explain why.

You will have your main Home Health Agency you're working for of course but what if your patient ends up sick and in the hospital? You do not get paid if that patient is in the hospital. So how will you get paid to pay your bills and etc? You have your second and third agency. You can ask all three of the agencies if they have anything available in the meantime until your patient is back home from the hospital. You will have more options this way. Majority of the time some agencies will try to send you to a case no one wants to work and they know at this point you're desperate to work. Well, if you have multiple agencies you can pick the best one that is right for you. Instead of being stuck with a case that is just horrible.

Majority of the patients get Physical Therapy, Speech Therapy and Occupational Therapy. These therapies can be done at patients' homes or in a facility.

Also this works if you're doing a three day twelve hour shift with one case, you have options to work another case for the remaining two or three days if you choose. Do you see how that works in your favor? Home Health agencies have its pros and cons. Let's get to it shall we.

<u>PROs of working Home Health</u>

1) You get to meet some nice people sometimes.
2) You gain a lot of skills which consist of Trach and Vent, G tube, PICC Lines and different machines to use and how they suit your patient.
3) Medical, vision and dental benefits are good for some home health agencies. While others are so high you will end up one of the nurses without any insurance at all. This is sad because nurses put in so many hours and hard work to assist in the proper care and treatment for their patient yet we are forgotten about a lot.
4) You meet other amazing nurses and it helps when you need someone that actually understands where you're coming from.
5) There's always something new to learn.
6) Majority of them use electronic documents.
7) You can get a case that is close to home if available.
8) One to one care versus One to twenty something patient ratio.
9) Raises for being an outstanding nurse.
10) Free classes to up your skills or memory on whatever it is you need.

Different Types of Home Health Cases

1.   CPS Cases

2.   The at home full time parent cases.

3.   The working parents cases.

4.   G - Tube Cases

5.   Trach patient cases

Chapter One

With being a nurse on a cps case, you have to have mental, physical and spiritual strength. It's very stressful at times. Basically the patient is taken away from the parents because CPS felt the safety of the child was in jeopardy. In some cases the parent is able to visit with the child either at a CPS office or at the current home patient resides.

Now this is where it can get complicated and even dangerous. If the parent has severe mental illness and not taking their medication things can really get out of hand. If the parent is on drugs or just simply not mature. Some of these parents will curse at you, threaten you and people involved with the child and at times might lead to physical assault. Hopefully it will not reach that point in your case.

Majority of the time you have to be aware of your surroundings and make sure you are always on point. The important person of course is yourself for you and your families safety but also your patients safety and well being. As a nurse you are the advocate for your patient. Remember the patient is obviously going through a lot and it can affect them mentally and physically. They Are confused and just don't know what exactly is going on but know something is not right.

So you should make sure you're okay and your patient is even better. This is where your compassion and empathy goes on high and expressed through nursing care and love. Some cases can get really bad and can be life threatening.
It's your decision on if you want to stay or seek another case.

With that being sad it can get better for some. Sometimes the biological parents get themselves together and eventually get their child back. With hard work and dedication it can happen but they just have to do what it takes to make it happen.

If you do decide to take a CPS case do remember why you became a nurse. No one said it will be easy. You will have some ups and downs with good and stressful cases. It's up to you to decide if you will be okay with working with a case like this. Do know if you do decide you want to, you are a vital part of the child's life.

If you leave, that will be a heartbreak for that child. At that point and time in their life, they need someone that will advocate for them and take the best care of the patient. You are very vital in their life and once they get used to you, they will adore you for a very long time. In some cases they get older and remember that nurse or nurses that were there for them in those very hard times in their life.

If you do decide to work a CPS case, Thank you for your hard work and dedication to what you do. You are really appreciated and one in a million. Thank you.

Chapter Two

What can I say? This type of case can be very difficult at times. You're probably wondering what I mean by this. Basically you're doing your nursing Duty with your patient and you have parents that are always home. Sometimes they could distract the patient from doing what they need to do via doctor's Orders. In other cases the parents try to get you to do something that is not in your nurse orders and you know you're not supposed to do that.

As a nurse we are all taught to do things that are ordered by a physician. If you do anything that's outside of that you could be held accountable and the worst thing that could happen is you lose your license. I'm sure you work hard for your license Blood Sweat and Tears as we all have done. In some of these cases you have to tell the parent that without an order you cannot administer certain medications or do certain things without it. Also you have to let your company know what is going on just in case anything happens they are aware of the situation and back you up.

With that being said you have to make sure that you do what is ordered and stay away from what is not ordered. If you do decide to do that parent a favor they will always want you to do that favor for them and if you guys end up on a bad note they could use that against you. I have seen and heard this done to some nurses and they have learned their lesson. They have learned that yes you might have a close relationship with the patient's family but if you do or you don't do as they want they will lie. They will try to get you to lose your license or your job.

Some people don't believe this happens, it actually does happen everyday in the medical field. So make sure please to only do what your order to do and yes have some sort of communication and relationship with the patient's family to let them know there's certain things that you are allowed to do and others you are not allowed to do. Once you stand up for yourself the parent will see and respect your decision. Some families will not respect your decision and try to do the things stated above. You have to be careful with some of these homes because they will do anything they can to get rid of you. It is ridiculous to see that people go out of their way to get you fired or to the extreme lose your license. But this is the world unfortunately we live in.

In some homes parents are a blessing. They're very helpful, kind and understanding. They understand that you're there to do your job and you love what you do. Of course you have to understand what the parents are thinking , this stranger is in my house taking care of my child so you have to build that trust with that parent. To let them know hey I am here yes but I am here for the patient and I'm going to give this patient the best care possible. Once you gain the trust of the parent / family everything will eventually fall into place. Do know they will always be wary of you because of all these videos and all of these horror stories of some nurses abuse mentally and physically their patients. So you have to be understanding on their part.

Once you build their trust and they see the daily routine that you have for the patient it will be good chemistry and communication between you both. Always make sure you document. Why do I say this, it doesn't matter if you're in home health, nursing home, assisted living, the hospital, travel nurse plain and simple you must document. Document and cover yourself of course and your company from any liability or any lies or so on and so forth. If you're with a patient for example and your patient is fine, respirations are good, make sure to document it at the end of shift also. At the end of your shift you give the oncoming nurse report. Within a few minutes of giving the report and you're on your way home that patient could decline and something could go wrong with the oncoming nurse.

Now if you did not document this information guess who's the blame for this?   In this nursing World / medical world they can hold you accountable for this. Why do I say this, for the simple fact that you did not document how you left the patient and they don't know what occurred at the end of your shift. I do know it takes some nurses time to finish documenting their day with the patient because there's so much that actually goes on.

But always remember to at least document that information to cover yourself as well as the company that you're working for. So at least it shows you had this documented at a certain time. Yes even if an oncoming nurse is with the patient at that time on her shift and something goes wrong that nurse could actually say the patient wasn't well on your shift. Yes they do have those types of nurses unfortunately in this world. This is why you have to be an advocate for yourself and your patient. Make sure you document.

Without your documentation guess what? It never happened. So word of advice, make sure you document. If it's a lot that you have to document and you normally go home and finish please at least document how you left the patient and reported to the oncoming nurse.   In some homes like I was explaining some parents could be really over you and pressure you to do things you're not supposed to do and that makes an environment very uncomfortable.

Knowing that you're going to someone's home to do what you're supposed to do as a nurse and someone is constantly hovering over you and constantly trying to tell you what to do can be very stressful. Yet there are some homes that the family is understanding and wants to get to know you.   Once you build that trust they fully understand and will let you do your job. They will not hover over you and they will not try to force or pressure you to do something that is not ordered by a physician.

So with that being said it's up to you to decide hey if you want to be in a household where the parent is home full-time.   You can decide if you want to stay with a household that the family is hovering over you or a family that actually understands and lets you do your job. I have heard many horror stories of people that have hovering parents and it makes their job miserable for the majority of their shift. I also heard some wonderful stories of full-time at home parents that are loving and caring and understandable.

So it's up to you if you want that full-time parent at home let the company know you do not mind. But if you do change your mind, let the company know that you prefer parents that are not home or just a different case due to the fact of being uncomfortable with those parents. Yes, it's about the patient but if you have someone constantly hovering over you and pressuring you it can make your job difficult.   It can make you and your patient uncomfortable. So that's something to think about if you want that full-time parent in the home sometimes they are helpful and sometimes they're not.

In some cases I've heard from other nurses that some parents are there but not there. If you get what I'm saying. basically they want you to do every and anything for that child but they do not want any involvement at all not even spending quality time with their child. They want to go out as they please and sometimes forget that you are not a babysitter. That's when your company comes into play and reminds them to reintegrate to that parent that you are there for patient needs only and nothing else.

Chapter 3

This is one of those cases that a lot of Home Health nurses which could be a LVN or RN rather have.   I have seen and heard nurses say they prefer to work at a home where the parents are not there.   The reason for this is all the facts from the last chapter.   It's unfortunate that a lot of nurses have been through the hovering parents and with some of the parents you understand the reason why.   But in a lot of the cases it can be very stressful to deal with on a daily basis.

That's why if you do get one of these cases that has working parents and you're able to concentrate and focus on your patient with no interruptions that's a blessing.   Cases like this are actually hard to come by but when you do get one you have to hold on to that case because other nurses are looking for this particular type of case.   You will have no interruptions, you're able to stay on the schedule for you and your patient. This will actually help your patients in the long run to get familiar with a set schedule.

You basically don't have to worry about anyone hovering over you, criticizing you or telling you what they want you to do for your patient. You will have a piece of mind knowing that you can do whatever that's ordered to maintain and make sure your patient is okay. You don't have to deal with a whole lot of family members coming over disrupting the order or schedule the patient is currently on.

If your patient does take a nap, you're able to get some very good documentation on what occurred so far and you won't be so behind in your charting. You are able to clean, maintain the patient's area to avoid infection and make sure the area is safe. There's not much to say on this part. But a lot of nurses prefer to have parents who actually go to work and let the nurse do their job.

So I'm going to leave it at this.   If you come across one of these cases and if you feel comfortable being with the patient by yourself then go for it. But if you do not feel comfortable in the house with the patient by yourself then you can ask about a case where the parents are home during the day.

Chapter 4

These are very common cases to work as a home health nurse. You can be an RN or LVN and work with a G-tube patient. Let me explain exactly what it means as a G-tube patient. It is Gastrointestinal tube patient. A gastrostomy tube also called G-tube is a tube inserted through the abdomen that delivers nutrition directly to the stomach. It's one of the ways doctors can make sure kids with trouble eating get the fluid and calories they need to grow.

Some gastrointestinal tubes deliver nutrition directly to the stomach or small intestine. They also could be used to deliver medications that are ordered by the doctor. This patient has to get proper care physically and also to maintain patency of the G-tube. As their nurse you have to make sure that it's still functioning, cleaned, flushed and whatever they are to receive via G-tube. Just make sure the patient receives what's ordered at the time ordered by the doctor. If there's any type of redness around the stoma site.

You have to document, treat it, call the G.I. doctor as well as the primary care physician. If this G-tube happens to come out , you as the nurse have to know exactly what it entails to keep the opening protected and not close. You have to know what to do in order to maintain and make sure the patient is okay. Some G tubes are changed every 6 months. You have to check to make sure it is functioning, it's in the right location and there's nothing wrong with this G-tube.

For every shift you have to verify placement, check and see the stoma which is the skin around the area is either regular skin color, some redness, break down the skin, or any other issue that may come about. Always remember to document what it is you see and what have you done to take care of the problem.

If you do not document it never happens. G- tube patients are the first ones nurses tend to get when they enter into Home Health Care. Some of the nurses learn how to work with tracheostomy patients. Majority of the time nurses are more comfortable working with these G-Tube patients rather than tracheostomy patients. Some of these patients are mobile and some are not mobile.

Chapter 5

A tracheotomy is a hole in the front of the neck into the windpipe. A tracheotomy tube is then inserted through the hole. The patient can then breathe on his or her own, or be ventilated through the tube. These tubes come in different sizes and types. It is always good to know what size they have and always have a size smaller available just in case. Majority of these patients have oxygen tanks and ventilators. Some of the patients need the oxygen throughout the day or just PRN. Some patients need their ventilator during the day 24/7 or just overnight to assist them with breathing.

Sometimes these cases can be very stressful because of the amount of care and need to make sure to maintain that trach.   In these cases they usually have a G-tube and a trach so you have two things you're working on. For Trach patients you get paid a little more because it's a trach patient. With G-tube patients you get paid a little less because it's just a G-tube you're working with versus working with actually two things. Some of these patients are bed-bound and some can actually walk around or utilize a wheelchair or Walker.

With these cases you definitely have to make sure you know exactly what you're doing. You're in their home with the family or the family is not there so you have to make sure you definitely know exactly what to do just in case the patient is not able to breathe. We have to know exactly what to do if the patient's trach comes out or the patient pulls out the trach. Some patients do pull out their trach unfortunately when they get upset.

Some home health agencies do offer a training class with them to help assist you and train you to answer any questions that's needed so you're able to take on a trach patient case. Other Home Health agencies will send you to training which will last an entire day to make sure you understand the importance of maintaining the opening of the trach, making sure the trach stays in place, making sure the stoma is clean and no skin breakdown. Some get scared to take care of these patients because a lot of the time they could be newborns with a trach.

This can be frightening to some nurses because the babies are so delicate. Sometimes patients are able to talk and majority of times they're not able to talk. In those cases there is a special speaking valve called a passy Muir valve that can be placed on a tracheostomy tube to improve speech even while on the ventilator.

Do always remember you are that patient's advocate so if they cannot speak you have to find a way to communicate with them and understand what they're trying to communicate to you. Some do sign language and some are able to write down what is needed if they cannot talk. Some of the patients actually cannot communicate at all so you have to find a way to understand and work with your patient. I actually worked with a patient that was not able to talk.   She learned sign language to be able to communicate. I learned sign language due to the patient. So I was able to understand and communicate with her. As a nurse you do what it takes to educate yourself and to make sure your patient is well taken care of. I know some sign language now so I'm happy about that.

Some advice

Whatever you're able to get certified in I suggest you do so.
I also suggest that you get some sort of experience in
med-surg, labor and delivery, and also mental health depending on
what you prefer. But do get some sort of experience in the hospitals.
Or clinics. It will test you and your skills to the Max and will be
very stressful but it will be beneficial in the long run.

Yes it's scary in the beginning because some of the nurses that
are well seasoned can be very mean, but do remember you were made
for this, you were born for this. You bust your butt to get to where
you are now. Don't ever let anyone make you feel otherwise. You will
not know every single thing. you will not remember everything
that you have learned this is why it's best you get your hands on

experience and take it to the next level. If you're comfortable with doing certain things and you rather stay there then that's your decision, no one is judging you. If you want to be a nurse that knows a little bit of everything or almost everything, take that advice and go for it. You can do it. I believe in you. You did everything you needed to do in nursing school to obtain your license. Welcome to the nursing world. The nursing world is not easy at all. It's just like school at times Blood Sweat and Tears. Is it worth it? yes it is. I wouldn't have it any other way.

I've learned so many things as being a nurse for years that I love what I do. At times don't get me wrong I sit and think oh my goodness what did I get myself into. Then I realized I was made for this, so therefore I'm going to continue to strive to be the best nurse that I could be. With that being said you go out there and be the best nurse that you can be for yourself. Do not hinder nor limit yourself from your true potential in this world. Nursing is hard but it is what we signed up for. You will have your many ups and your many downs but don't you give in and don't you quit. That dark

CLOUD WOULD NOT BE AROUND FOREVER. IF YOU REALLY ENJOY WHAT YOU DO AND LOVE WHAT YOU DO, THE PATIENTS CAN TELL. THE LOOK ON THEIR FACES OF THANKING YOU, ADMIRING YOU FOR DOING WHAT YOU DO AND PUTTING UP WITH THEIR MESS SOMETIMES IS ALL THAT YOU NEED TO SEE AND WITNESS. THIS SHOWS YOU HOW MUCH YOU'RE APPRECIATED AND SOMETIMES YOU'RE NOT APPRECIATED BUT GUESS WHAT THE ONES ACTUALLY APPRECIATE YOU OUTWEIGHS THE NEGATIVE ONES.

DO NOT HESITATE TO GET MORE KNOWLEDGE ON YOUR CRAFT. BE BETTER, DO BETTER AND YOU WILL SEE SO MUCH MORE. THANK YOU GUYS FOR TAKING THE TIME TO READ MY BOOK. I HOPE YOU ENJOYED IT.

How to survive working Home Health Nursing.

The End

Repeat Prescriptions

When working within a care setting where the people cared for require ongoing medication often there will be a facility for repeat prescriptions built into a prescription. These can be in batches which will mean that there will not be a significant build-up of medication which may go out of date but will also give the doctor a chance to review the situation of the patient at intervals to ensure the medication is working properly and not causing any adverse side effects. A repeat prescription should be filled prior to the previous prescription being completed to allow continuity of treatment.

When arranging a repeat prescription the following steps should be followed:

1. Establish what medicines are nearing the end of their cycle
2. Contact the GP's surgery to arrange a new prescription. Be aware that this could take up to 28 days and may require a visit to the GP.
3. When the prescription arrives check it against the old MAR chart to ensure there are no errors in dosage or medication. Contact the surgery immediately if there are any issues.
4. Lodge the prescription with the pharmacist ensuring it is completed correctly (as described above). Once received back from the pharmacist check the medication again for any errors and report it immediately if there are any errors
5. Enter the medication onto the MAR chart making note of any balances to be carried forward from previous months. This must be checked by a second member of staff to ensure accuracy and both staff members should sign and date the chart.
6. Store the medication in a secure trolley or cabinet. Only those responsible for the administration of medication should have access to this store.

Once these steps have been completed the medication can be used as instructed and any leaflets should also be read. The carer also needs to watch out for side effects as normal.

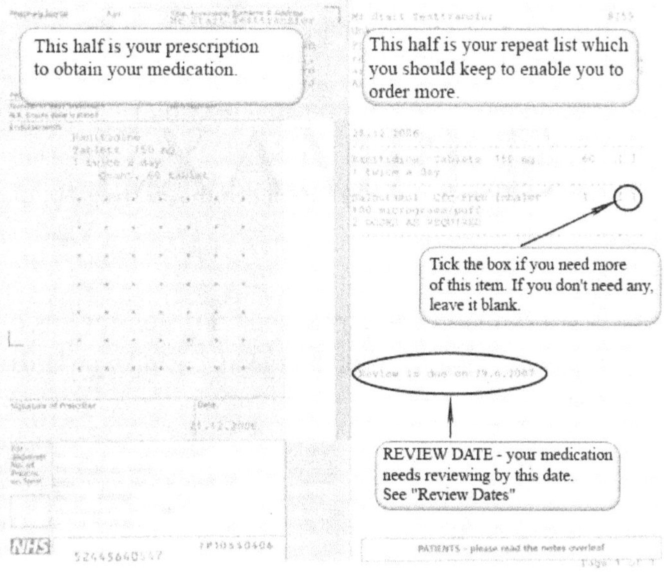

Mental Capacity Act (2005)

This Act was fully implemented in 2007 and replaced part 7 of the Mental Health Act 1983. This also replaced the ENDURING POWER Of ATTORNEY ACT 1985.

Within this act neglect was criminalized i.e. a person accused of neglecting another individual will have broken the law and can be dealt with within the criminal justice system. This act will help and offer guidance to people who can make some decisions about their treatment, and live a mainly independent life, but who may need help with some other aspects of their being – such as being able to live independently but needing help to cook hot meals. This act also incorporates 'advanced decisions' which is when someone with mental capacity decides that they do not want a particular type of treatment if they lack capacity in the future; a doctor must respect this decision.

The act is underpinned by 5 key principles:

- An individual is assumed to be capable unless proven otherwise
- An individual should be supported to make their own decisions
- An individual has the right to make unorthodox decisions
- The individual's best interests must be the focus
- Any intervention should be as unrestrictive as possible

As shown above all adults are presumed to have sufficient capacity to decide their own medical treatment unless proven that this capacity is impaired. There several reasons this ability could be impaired, including but not limited to:

- Mental health conditions such as schizophrenia, bi-polar disorder or dementia
- Serious learning difficulties
- Conditions which may cause drowsiness, confusion or loss of consciousness
- Intoxication caused by drugs or alcohol

Additionally, in order for someone to be proven capable of making their own decision they need to show that they:

- Understand the information about the medication and their condition that they have been given
- Are able to remember that information
- Are able to use that information as part of their decision-making process
- Are able to communicate their decision by talking, using sign-language or other clear means

It is important to remember that not being "capable" of making a decision about medication is not the same as actively choosing not to take medication that is generally considered in their best interest or making a decision about their medication that may seem irrational. An example of this is the difference between someone with dementia refusing to take medicine they need for their diabetes compared with someone who is medically capable refusing the most efficient medicine for their treatment because it had been tested on animals during its development.

This can be particularly difficult for the carer as they are generally the person responsible for administering the medication. Situations such as these are covered under the guidelines of the Mental Capacity Act 2005, allowing decisions to be made on behalf of an individual if they are unable to do so, or stipulating that the decisions of the person, though seemingly unwise, may not be ignored because they are of sound mind. If the carer finds themselves in this position the five principals above can be used as a guide.

In order to comply with these principles the following advice can be used:

- Give clear information about the choices that are available to them.
- Ensure information is given in context (eg in the setting where the activity will be).
- Arrange the environment in a way that helps better communication.
- Choose a time when they are more receptive (when they are more lucid)
- Give the information in a way that the person can understand.
- Monitor their response, and get feedback on what is happening to gauge their understanding.

In some cases people can be considered capable to decide about some aspects of their treatment but not about other aspects. For example, a person with severe learning difficulties may be capable of deciding about their day-to-day treatment but be incapable of understanding the complexities of their long-term treatment.

Also, some people with certain health conditions may have periods when they are capable, and periods when they are not, such as the early stages of dementia. In such circumstances, a person can make a "living will" or a statement of "advanced decisions", stating how they would like to be treated, or not treated, in the future if their capacity is diminished. Under the Mental Health Act "advanced decision" are legally binding upon every one providing care for the individual unless the person is being held under the Mental Health Act.

In cases where a person has been deemed unable of making decisions for themselves a "decision team" will be put together to make decisions in the best interest of the person and will include people such as care staff, a GP, family members, a social worker and an independent advocate.

This Act enshrines into law in the UK the fundamental rights and freedoms contained in the European Convention on Human Rights. These rights not only impact matters of life and death, they also affect the rights you have in your everyday life: what you can say and do, your beliefs, your right to a fair trial and other similar basic entitlements. Under this act people have the responsibility to respect other people's rights.

Basic human rights of life are:
- the right to life
- freedom from torture and degrading treatment
- freedom from slavery and forced labour
- the right to liberty
- the right to a fair trial
- the right not to be punished for something that wasn't a crime when you did it
- the right to respect for private and family life
- freedom of thought, conscience and religion, and freedom to express your beliefs
- freedom of expression
- freedom of assembly and association
- the right to marry and to start a family
- the right not to be discriminated against in respect of these rights and freedoms
- the right to peaceful enjoyment of your property
- the right to an education
- the right to participate in free elections
- the right not to be subjected to the death penalty

If any of these rights and freedoms are breached, the person has a right to an effective solution in law, even if the breach was by someone in authority, such as police officer or doctor.

Right to Refuse - A fundamental part of our human rights is the right to refuse medication. As stated previously, as long as a person has the mental capacity to make an informed decision and they do so voluntarily then their decision must be respected regardless of the likely outcome. A qualification to this is that if a person requests a treatment that a healthcare professional does not believe is in the best interest of that person then the healthcare professional is under no obligation to provide it.

Right to Privacy - As a key part of our human rights the respect for a private life means that confidentiality is essential when looking after a person. A carer will have access to intimate and personal details about the person they look after through the nature of their work. It is a priority to preserve their confidentiality and not discuss their medication, condition or any part of their personal information with anyone else **without their express permission**. Any person who breaks that confidentiality will be held accountable.

Remember not to make assumptions about the relationship of the family member or friend – it is not always appropriate to openly discuss individual cases.

Check if the individual has given permission to talk to them.

Right to Self-Determination - As already discussed in the Mental Capacity section, as long as someone has sufficient mental capacity they have the right to make their own decision about what treatment they receive. Implicit in this right is the principle of "patient consent" whereby a patient must give express permission before any medical treatment is carried out and there cannot be any assumption that permission has been given on the part of the person administering medication. The type of the treatment is not important and can range from a finger prick test to organ transplant. This principle is enshrined in international law which reflects the central position consent plays in the ethics of medicine.

Consent must be:
1. **Voluntary** (and not a result of pressure or coercion by other)
2. **Informed** (and based on the whole facts, including what is involved, what benefits and risks there are, what alternatives are available and what will happen if the treatment is refused)

Where the person is unable to fulfil both of these criteria a decision team will make a decision based on their best interest and in these circumstances **only** consent will not be required.

We all have the right to decide what happens to us and when,
this is our Human Right.

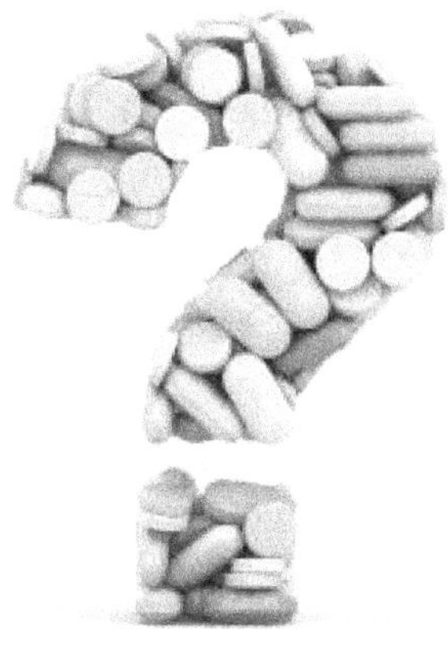

Probably the most important thing that a carer can do for a person in their care is ensure that they are safe and free from harm.

> **"Abuse is a violation of an individual's human and civil rights by any other person or persons"**
> *(No Secrets Department of Health 2000)*

People in care are, by virtue of the fact that they need to be looked after, very vulnerable to abuse. This is because, as their mental and physical abilities deteriorate, they become more dependent on others and less able to speak up for themselves.

It is important that policies and procedures exist in every professional care situation and that staff should be trained in recognizing the signs of abuse and how to report incidents of, or suspicions about, abuse taking place.

With regard to medication, there are some forms of abuse that specifically apply:

1. ***INSTITUTIONAL ABUSE****: an organization imposing rigid and insensitive routines; unskilled, intrusive or invasive interventions; or an environment allowing inadequate privacy or physical comfort*
   a. Lack of, or poorly followed, care plans can mean that a person's medication is not at its optimal situation. For instance, not reviewing a person's condition regularly enough may lead to their medication not being suitable anymore or an increase in side effects
   b. Rigid structures with no opportunity to individualized arrangements will mean that if a person would like to try alternative treatments they would not be able to.
2. ***NEGLECT AND/OR ACTS OF OMMISSION:*** *intentionally or unintentionally ignoring medical or physical care needs*
   a. This could lead to untreated physical illness
   b. Repeated infections
3. ***CHEMICAL ABUSE****; over-use of medication to control or manage their behaviour.*
   a. Constantly appearing drowsy
   b. Repeated falls
   c. Low staff / patient ratios or poor management
   d. Lack of medication reviews

Remember: Over-medication in people is a form of abuse.

Abuse is not always deliberate or malicious but instead can result from;

- Poor understanding of an individual's needs and abilities
- Poor understanding of aggression as a form of communication
- Stress through lack of staff or time
- Lack of organisational support and training

CARE IN THE HOME

Abuse that is taking place in a private home is often harder to identify as the carer will only go in at certain times. In these circumstances the risk of harm and abuse can be heightened due to a number of reasons;

- Stress on the person doing the bulk of the caring
- Unsuitable accommodation/environment
- Lack of knowledge as to help available
- Over protectiveness due to fear of what might happen to a loved one resulting in choices not being available

DON'T IGNORE IT!

Every organization should be acting with the best interests of their clients at heart and so should welcome reports of any situation which goes against this. Staff should be made aware that they encourage whistle blowing and will act to restore the best practice if anything is reported, without penalising the person who reported the abuse.

If someone has disclosed to you that they are being abused, or you suspect abuse is taking place, you must inform your line manager.
If that is not possible, contact CQC, social services or the police.

Remember to record and document everything, including your name, the date and time.

The approach to care over the past 20 years has changed. The needs of the cared-for-person were generally ignored, and they were failed in terms of meeting their specific, individual requirements. This is because there was a general negative culture of a sense of hopelessness about looked after people. The value of the person was disregarded and the care process was managed according to what was convenient for the care provider rather than according to the whole needs of the person.

There have, however, been significant changes in the care of people. There has been a shift in emphasis from focusing upon a person's losses and dependencies, to an appreciation of their remaining strengths and abilities. Additionally there has been an emphasis placed on the "personhood" of the cared for person and a recognition that each person has many unique and individual needs.

According to the Government's National Service Framework for Older People[2], it should be the aim of care providers to ensure that older people are treated as individuals and they receive appropriate and timely packages of care which meet their needs as individuals. One of the ways of achieving this is to implement the Person-Centred Care Approach. This involves:

Listen to the person	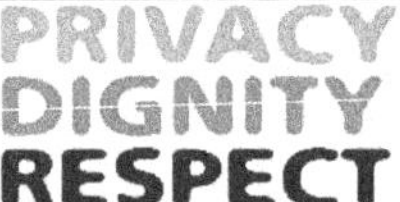 Show the person respect by allowing them to keep their dignity and privacy
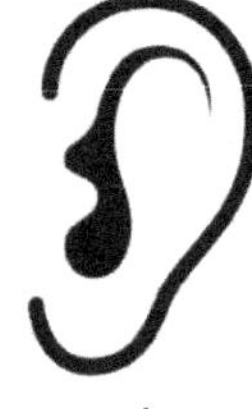 Recognise individual differences and specific needs including cultural and religious differences	Enable the person to make informed choices. Involve them in all decisions about their needs and care 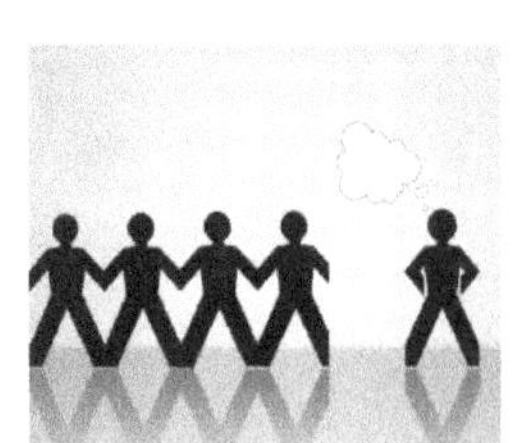

In terms of care of those being looked after the following criteria would show successful application of the Person-Centred Approach:

- Promoting the value and individuality
- Seeking to understand looked after people's personal motivations
- Treating looked after people with respect and dignity
- Listening to what looked after people have to say
- Promoting choice, independence and empowerment for people

GOOD PRACTICE MEANS MEETING THE NEEDS OF THE WHOLE PERSON

A Person-Centred Approach to providing care and support is as important for the people who receive services (and their family or significant others) as it is to staff. The emphasis should always be on the person as an individual and their unique qualities, likes, dislikes, wishes and their defining characteristics. People who are being looked after have the same rights as all people. Care and support services should build on individual strengths and abilities to maximize and promote independence. Services should enable people to feel valued and safe.

The use of medication should be a key part of a Person-Centred assessment and regular reviews would need to be carried out to ensure the effectiveness of this medication and how it fits in with the whole person care. This means:

- A full assessment is carried out prior to any service being offered and reviews are carried out on an ongoing basis
- Detailed records to show that the individual is fully involved in the assessment process and the language used in the assessment is appropriate to all parties
- Religious and cultural needs are fully understood and met
- The well-being of the individual is actively promoted
- The care plans are laid out in such a way that they may be used as communication, recoding and evaluation tools
- Named carers or key workers are matched appropriately to the individual
- Relatives and significant others are made to feel involved and supported

Please see our course book Person-Centred Planning (06PC) for more information.

With the best will in the world carers may be unaware that their actions have a negative impact on a person in care. The best way to avoid this is to get to know the person in care so that they can be seen as an individual who can make their own choices. It can be easy for degrading and dangerous stereotypes to creep into an attitude about people with care, such as the fact that the need to be treated like babies. It can become as though the care is done **to** them and not **for** them, reducing their power of self-determination, a basic human right.

When caring for people in a care setting remember:

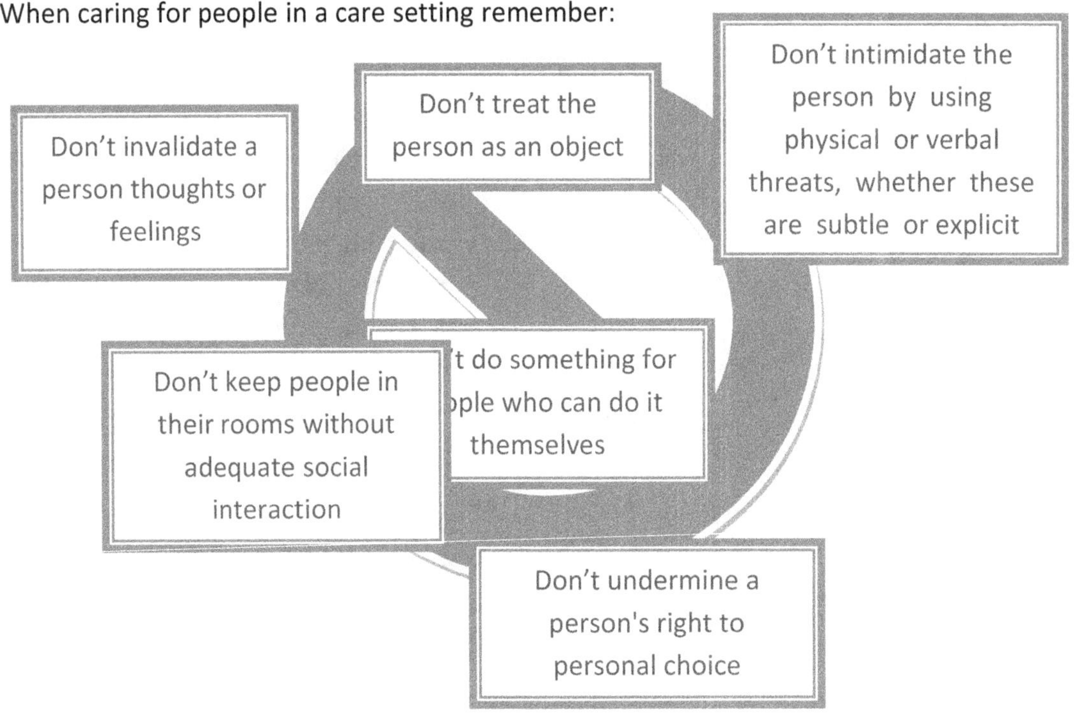

Instead the role of a carer should be to provide:

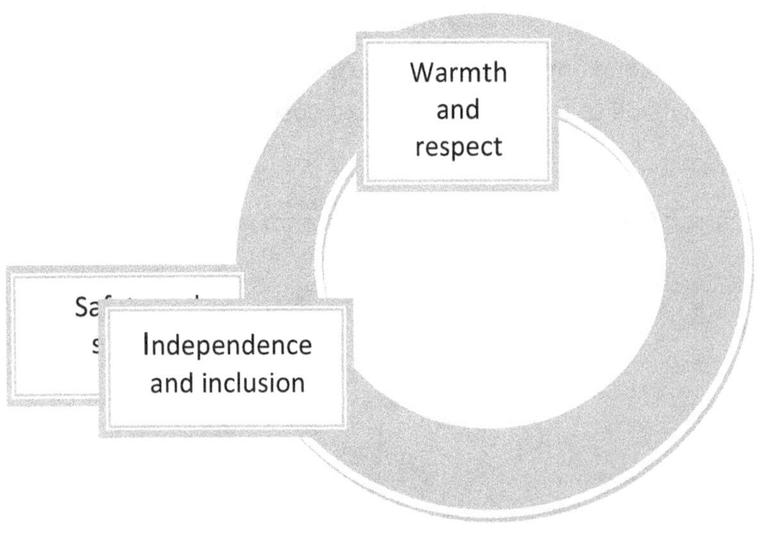

The added benefit of getting to know a client really well is that it is easier to spot when there are strange effects or behaviours that may be a side effect of some of their mediation, allowing steps to be taken to remedy the situation.

Whatever illness a person has it is vital that they be included as much as possible in discussion about their care. There are three key reasons for this: it is a fundamental part of the Person-Centred Approach, it is key to ensuring the client's best interests are kept at heart, and it is the best way for the individual to retain as much control over their life quality as possible.

This begins by ensuring that they are engaged with the conversation with the GP and, in as far as possible, the carer or someone else does not speak for them. It also means that their opinion about what medication they wish to take and in what form should be listened to. Finally, any comments they have about how the programme of treatment is going should be carefully noted and taken into account. It is important to remember to keep the person taking the medicine at the centre of the discussion.

REMEMBER - *Regular reviewing and assessments will be a vital part of the role of the carer.*

Assessments and reviews will be required when:
There is change in a looked after person's physical or mental health or lasting or adverse side effects are noted
The looked after person requests a review
When a review is requested by significant others, such as family and social worker

Residential/Nursing Home Care Plan

NHS No:
H&SC No:

Surname:

Telephone:

First Name:

Title:

Address:

Persons stated preferences e.g. likes, dislikes and routines etc:

Effective Care Co-ordination ☐

Manual Handling ☐

Medication ☐

Please State:

Other ☐

If No: State Reason below:

Separate Risk Assessment Completed:

Smoking ☐

Is the Service User Satisfied with the Care Plan? Yes ☐ No ☐

Date Care Plan Given/Sent to Carer:

Care Plan End Date:

Date Care Plan Given/Sent to Service User:

Care Plan Start Date:

Date:

Designation:

Date Care Plan Sent to Other Care Providers:

Name:

Signed by Assessor:

As a minimum standard, care and support will be reviewed annually. If the person's needs change before the next review please contact the following number:

Reviewing

Care Plan Review Date:

23/10/07

According to the Medicines (labelling) Regulations 1975 as amended, medicines can only be administered from a container with a pharmacist's label which complies with the regulations. An example of one of these labels, with an explanation of its component parts, can be seen below.

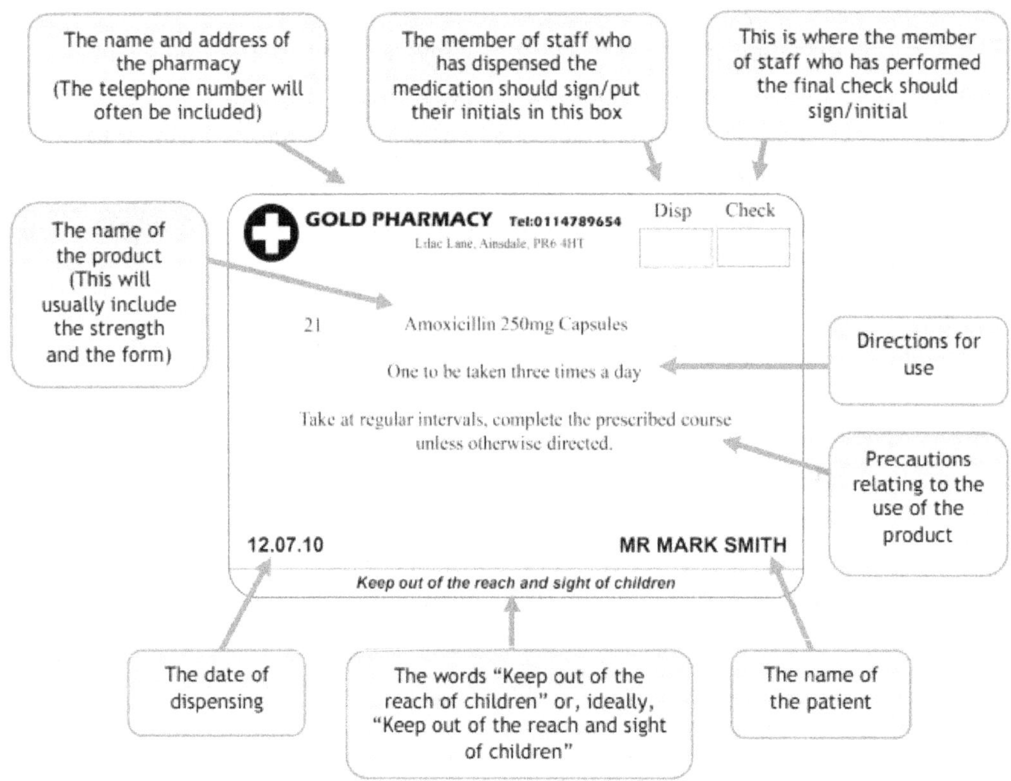

These labels include various types of information and in addition to those mentioned above could include the name and address of the patient's doctor, and the date of birth and NHS number of the patient.

As already discussed there are several ways that medicine can be dispensed; bottles, boxes and blister packs, in the form of tablets (soluble and non-soluble), capsules, liquid, inhalers, eye drops, creams, patches or through other methods directly into the body to name a few.

A pharmacist may also wish to assess the individual needs of the person to decide the best form to dispense the medication for them and not disadvantage them in anyway. For instance, is it more appropriate for medication to be dispensed in a compliance aid blister pack, a container or as a liquid? This approach is in compliance with the Equality Act 2010.

This act replaced most of the previous Disability Discrimination Act 1995. Under this act, disabled people cannot be discriminated against in respect of:

- Employment
- Education
- Access to goods, facilities and services
- Buying or renting land or property

It also incorporated the 2005 Act which amended or extended existing provisions in the DDA 1995 including;

- Making it unlawful for operators of transport vehicles to discriminate against disabled people
- Making it easier for disabled people to rent property and for tenants to make disability – related applications
- Making sure that private clubs with 25 or more members cannot keep disabled people out, just because they have a disability
- Extending protection to cover people who have HIV, cancer and multiple sclerosis from the moment it is diagnosed
- Ensuring that discrimination law covers all the activities of the public sector
- Requiring public bodies to promote equality of opportunity for disabled people

Health and Social Care Act (2012)

This act forms an umbrella under which all vulnerable people in whatever care setting are protected. It replaces the previous CARE STANDARDS ACT 2000 which replaced the Registered Homes Act 1984.

The Act follows the National Care Standards Commission (NCSC) which later became the Commission for Social Care Inspection (CSCI) and now is the Care Quality Commission (CQC)

The government introduced National Minimum Standards and established the General Social Care Council (GSCC) for England and the Care Council for Wales. These work towards raising the standards of practice through codes of conduct and practice.

The Act requires that any agency supplying care to a person within their own home (domiciliary) must be registered.

Control of Substances Hazardous to Health Regulations (1999) – (COSHH)

The primary function of this set of requirements is to protect people from the effects of potential dangerous substances. It makes it a responsibility of employers to take reasonable measures to protect their employees from harm they may receive from these substances while at work. But the COSHH was also developed as a guide on how to safely control the use of hazardous substances to reduce the risk of potential harm they may cause.

When it comes to medication, carers must be aware that, while it is the responsibility of employer to ensure safety around hazardous substances, it is also incumbent upon the employee to play an active role in the safe handling of medication for the benefit of all.

Practically this means:

- Knowing and understanding the various roles and responsibilities of those in the work place as well as those involved in prescribing, dispensing, administering and disposing of medication.
- Knowing and adhering to the policies and procedures of the work place, particularly with regard to recording and management of medication.
- Carefully reading any information relating to medication so that they understand the nature of the medication and any ramifications of its misuse.
- Remaining observant and vigilant throughout the medication process to ensure everything is as it should be.

National Service Framework for Older People

A National Service Framework (NSF) for older people (aged over 55) was published by the Department of Health in 2001. It is a 10 year framework for improving the health and social care of older people in England. It looks at how best to diagnose, assess and treat older people, as well as developing an integrated mental health service between local authorities and independent healthcare providers.

National Minimum Standards

The Department of Health has laid out a set of minimum standards for people over 65 in care. These National Minimum Standards for the care of older people in care homes are detailed in the "Care Homes for Older People; National Minimum Standards – Care Homes Regulations 3rd Edition (2000)" document. It provides a set of set of standards which must be achieved as well designating an individual who is responsible for ensuring these are met.

With regard to providing medication to people in care settings the National Minimum Standards require that the registered person should put into place a policy which describes how the medication should be handled in all of the following categories:

- Receipt
- Recording
- Storage
- Handling
- Administration
- Disposal

This will promote the safety and well-being individuals being cared for and makes staff aware of safe practices

Accordingly the Procedures and Policies of a nursing home should be carefully prepared to ensure they are practical and useful, they should be effectively communicated to both staff and service users and they should be reviewed from time to time to ensure they are kept up to date and adapted when needed.   Good practice is to write a set of policies and procedures that are unique to the workplace to which they apply, so that they are able to guide the employee through the use of medication from ordering to disposal, covering all the points mentioned above. Staff need to ensure that they familiarise themselves with the policies and procedures BEFORE dealing with any clients and that they are informed of any changes that occur subsequently.

The Home will have many policies and procedures to help in the event of an incident. All care staff should familiarise themselves with the information as it is there to protect and guide everybody.

P&Ps help carers in their daily tasks because it lets them:

- know what to expect and what is expected of them
- know what to do when certain events arise
- know where to go to find out more
- have a effective guide for working alongside clients and their families
- provide guidance when faced with an ethical dilemma

If carers are not aware of an organisations policies and procedures, or choose to disregard them, they run the risk of:

- Working differently to everyone else and therefore not working as a team
- Not using safe systems at work and as a consequence putting themselves and the individual they care for at risk
- Not knowing or helping to achieve organizational objectives
- Appearing unprofessional or presenting the organization in an unprofessional way

If a carer is unsure where the Policies and Procedures document is kept or does not understand any of the information, they must address this immediately with their manager who will be more than happy to help.

Many of a Home's policies will be derived from legislation or regulations. One such set of policies relates to the safety of the employees and service users in a home.

Requires the employer and the employee to take responsibility for health and safety whilst carrying out work. The act requires employers to provide a safe working environment and supply any equipment required to carry out the role i.e. personal protective equipment. It also safeguards the person with service users by ensuring they are not put at risk of harm whilst using the service.

The **PPEWR** advises on the selection of personal protective equipment and clothing worn or held by people at work to protect them against risks to their health and safety. PPE should only be considered after risk assessment when the risk from a specific hazard cannot be controlled effectively in any other way.

Like the COSHH, the Health and Safety Act and the PPEWR were established as guidance for both employers and employees in creating a work place that is safe and protects well-being. It makes both employers and employees responsible for one another's health and safety, and both employers and employees in turn are responsible for residents and visitors.

Additionally there is a duty on every employer to "ensure as far as is reasonably practicable the health, safety and welfare at work of all his employees" and that they "Conduct [their] undertakings in such a way as to ensure so far as is reasonably practicable, those persons not in [their] employment who may be affected thereby are not exposed to risks to their health or safety"

As an example some of the policies that may exist in a care home are:

- The employer will provide the correct equipment for any known risk staff may have while handling medicines, to reduce the risk of harm. This may include gloves, aprons, washing facilities and spillage kits or sharps disposal containers. *[This is a requirement under the legislation above]*
- Medicines should not be touched and extra precautions (for example, wearing gloves) must be taken for certain medicines that may cause harm if advertently handled, such as steroid creams.
- All creams and ointments should be applied using gloves to reduce both the risk of cross-contamination and also the possibility of harm to staff.
- Always wash hands thoroughly before starting a medicine round.
- Never undertake a medicine round without referring to the MAR chart while doing so. This should always be referred to before the administration or an application of any medicine.
- Have current drug information readily available, so it is possible to confirm a dose or understand why the medicine is being administered or to check for the side effects before actually administering it.

As can be seen below there are many people involved in the care of a person who is looked after but the person requiring care must be at the centre of the circle in accordance with the current Person-Centred approach to care and for the best outcomes for the person. The outside ring represents the connection these people have with each other as well as the person in need of care.

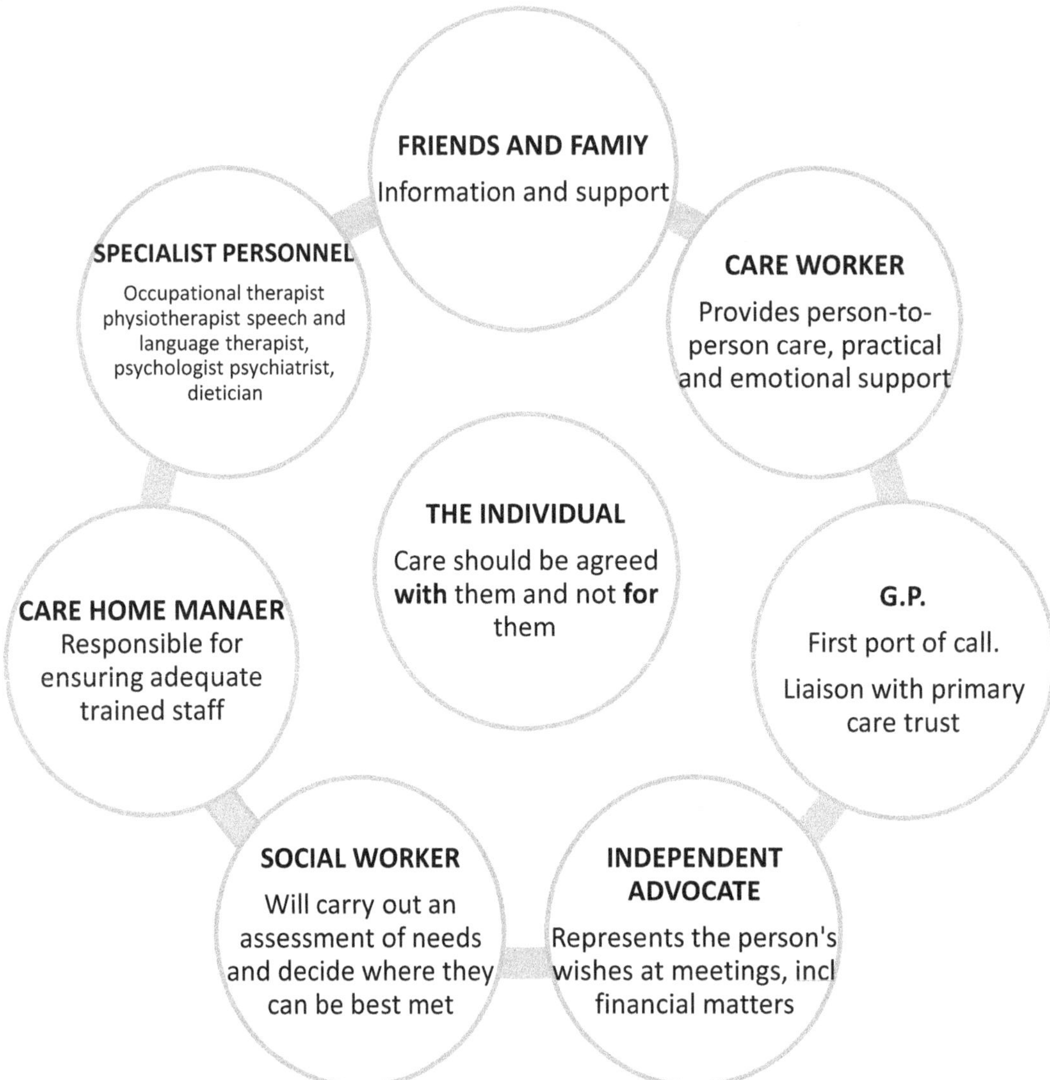

Those particularly involved with medication are:

- The GP who prescribes the medication
- The Pharmacist who dispenses the medication
- The Care Home Manager who is responsible for the medication from the time it is received from the Pharmacist until the time it is disposed of.
- The Care Worker is responsible for recording the usage of the medication, administering it and monitoring any adverse reaction due to it.
- The individual for whom the medication it is intended as, ultimately, for their benefit.

Roles and responsibilities may be divided up within the care workers of a home. For instance one person may be responsible for collecting prescriptions from a pharmacist and logging them in while another may have the responsibility of administering the medication to the people who are looked after in the home.

It is important that these separate roles are respected as crossing boundaries, even it is with the best intention of helping a colleague, may lead to errors or omissions which could end up causing harm to someone who is being looked after.

Care homes that also include a nursing facility will have clear separations as to who is responsible for controlling the medication. In homes where nursing is not provided, however, all staff must complete accredited training to ensure they fully understand the administration of medication, including a basic understanding of how medicines are used, how they work, what records must be kept and what to do in the event of a problem.

Ultimately, medication should only be handled by a competent fully trained member of staff. Any concerns about the handling and administration of medication in the care home should be reported to the line manager immediately.

Access to Health Records (1990)

This Act defines who may see medical records. The individual may see their own medical records but no one else may see them without permission from that individual. This includes next of kin and friends.

This Act governs the storage and processing of personal data held in manual records and on computers. Under this act, rights are protected by forcing organizations to follow proper and sound practices, known as data protection principles (DPP).

The data protection Act contains 8 principles which state that all data must be:

1. Processed fairly and lawfully
2. Obtained and used only for specified and lawful purposes
3. Adequate, relevant and not excessive
4. Accurate, and where necessary, kept up to date
5. Kept for no longer than necessary
6. Processed in accordance with the individuals rights and available for access to those individuals
7. Kept secure
8. Transferred only to countries that offer adequate data protection

EFFECTIVE RECORDING

As previously seen, one of the roles of a care worker is the recording of the receipt, distribution and disposal of medication. There are several things to consider when making records.

Keeping accurate and up to date records about a person being looked after is essential and an integral part of the carer's role. It is important for monitoring both the progress of their condition as well as the overall health and well-being.

Setting up suitable procedures can assist in ensuring excellent record keeping. Instructions on how to remain objective (avoid bias or personal opinions), when and how records should be taken, and what to include, should be made clear to everyone who has dealings with the person.

COMMON PROBLEMS WITH RECORDING TO WATCH OUT FOR

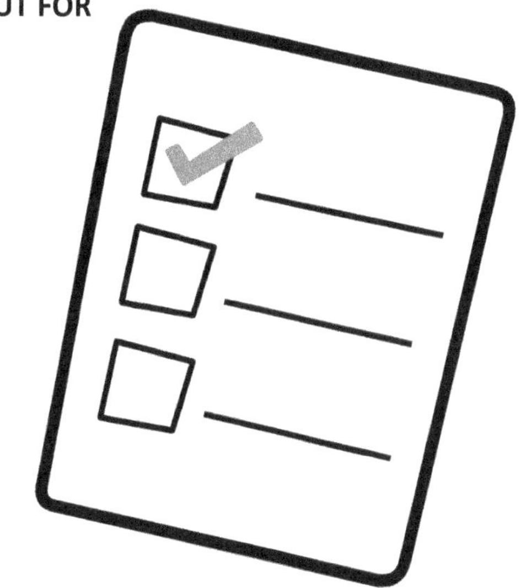

- Inappropriate language
- Lack of confidentiality
- Irrelevance
- Lack of objectivity
- Not fact based
- Not succinct (too long)
- Poor format
- Not written for sharing (code words etc)
- Not used as an analysis tool
- Illegible (poor handwriting)
- Not Person-Centred
- Lack of user involvement

*The best solution for all of these issues is to always remember the
reason that the records are being kept:*
TO PROVIDE THE BEST CARE POSSIBLE FOR THE INDIVIDUAL CONCERNED.

National Minimum Standards – Standard 9.3 (care homes for older people)
The above Standard requires that a record be kept of all medicines that are received, administered or leave the care home or go for disposal. This is done to prevent any mishandling. The registered person is responsible for keeping records of receipt, administration and disposal of medication.

The most common form of complying with this Standard is the MAR chart, which is an official record of administration to each individual and can be used as evidence in a court of law, all records must be kept up to date and accurate.

All information on a MAR chart must be printed or hand written in indelible ink. Sticking labels on is not permitted as they can be removed or transferred to another sheet. They may also cover up information that might have been needed and now cannot be seen.

The information on a MAR chart should contain:

- Name of the individual
- Name and address of the home
- Any allergies (if none write 'none known')
- Start date of the MAR chart
- Sequential page numbers (1 of 2, 2 of 2)
- Name, strength, dosage and formulation of medicine
- Quantity of medicine received and date
- Signature of two members of staff receiving the medication

The current medicine regime of new Service Users should be carefully checked to ensure all their medication is correct. This check is done according to the:

- discharge prescription from the hospital
- repeat prescription brought in by an individual
- pre-admission assessment by another health care professional

If this information is unavailable contact their G.P. Do not rely on an individual's word on what medication they are taking if they have no written confirmation to support it.

If a service user dies whilst in the care home all medication and records must be kept for 7 days as a coroner may wish to see them in the event of an unexplained or suspicious death.

When it comes to administering (or "giving") medication there are several things to remember.

1. Always remember to **wash your hands** before and after dealing with any medication or treatments for your service user.

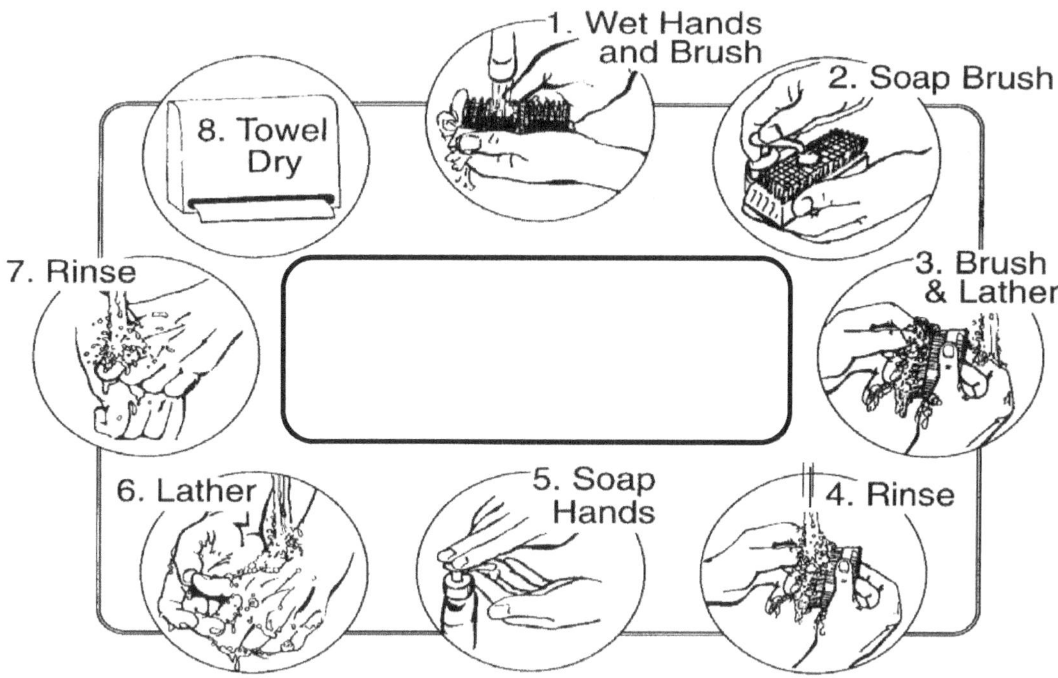

2. **Always read the label**. Full directions of how a doctor requires the medication to be administered or used should be specified on the prescription so that the pharmacist can label it as the doctor has intended.

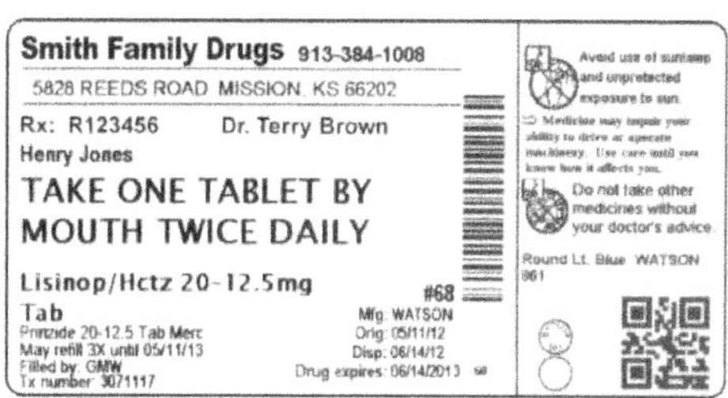

You must never divert from these instructions. Information leaflets will come with all medication including the blister packs if they do not, you can and should request them from the pharmacist who dispensed that medication.

Ensure the information on the label is correct and do not administer the medicine if it is not.

3. Ensure there is **agreement**. This is involves "compliance" and "concordance" where:

> ○ **Compliance** *means that the carer and the services user are in agreement about the administering and taking of that medication.*
>
> ○ **Concordance** *means that a health care professional and the service user have an agreement regarding their medication, it will also show a clear record of what they understand about their treatment, medication and if they want to take it.*

Good concordance will result in good compliance, for example a service user may not be in concordant with their medication because a certain prescribed medication that they take may make them feel unwell so then this leads to the service user not wishing to take their medication this results in poor compliance.

If such a situation occurs you must inform your manager and record your findings.

When you administer you must ensure that:
- The right individual receives
- The right medication
- In the right dose
- At the right time
- Through the right route

4. Ensure that the correct service use has been **identified** to make sure that the right medication is given to the right individual. There are simple checks that can be done:
    - Ask the service user their name (remember you may have two service users with the same name)
    - Ask a senior member of staff for help
    - Insert an identification page; this will have a photo of the service user on it.
    - Check the room number

In cases of mistaken identity report this immediately to a manager who will implement the home's policies and procedures for such an incident.
It is good practice for the carer to be familiar with this policies and procedures as well.

5. Maintain a list of **care staff who administer medication**. This list should also make it easy to identify the initials of each person who administers medication assisting in the recognition of each administer in the event of an error, incident or just for future reference.

Never sign for a medication before you have administered it.

Administration of medication is how medication can be given to a person and the Routes of Administration refers to the ways that medication can be introduced into the body. There are many different routes by which medication can be administered and the medical professional will decide on the best of these based on the speed of the absorption and the circumstances of the patient. Care staff should be aware of all of these and training is essential before any drugs are administered.

Below is a description of the various ways that medication can be given to a person:

Enteral

Medication absorbed though the digestive tract which includes pills, capsules or liquid taken by mouth (ingested orally), dissolved beneath the tongue (sublingual) or in the form of a suppository in the rectum. Absorption is slow and cannot be used if vomiting is occurring.

Mucosal

Medications are administered via the nasal mucosa, or bronchioles through inhalation of an aerosol. Vaginal administration of a medication is also considered mucosal.

Percutaneous

Medications are absorbed directly through the skin to the blood stream. Some hormone replacements are administered by patches that are absorbed slowly and evenly.

Parenteral

Parenteral refers to any non-oral means of administration but is generally interpreted to mean injecting a drug directly into the body, including into a vein (intravenous), muscle (intramuscular), an artery (intrarterial), the abdominal cavity (intraperitoneal), the heart (intracardiac), directly into bone marrow (intraosseous), just below the surface of the skin (transdermal), via a tube usually in the nose or mouth (endotracheal) or into the fatty tissue beneath the skin (subcutaneous). The speed of absorption varies but is faster than oral administration and is used when more complete and faster absorption is needed. It is unlikely that a carer will need to perform any of these procedures but they may be required to care for someone who has had one of these procedures.

Topical

This means creams, ointments and gels that are administered directly to the skin.

Instillation

Medication that is delivered one drop at a time, into to the ears, eyes or nose.

There are, of course, variations on many of these delivery methods, such as intravenous injections being given form via an intravenous tube but these will be predominantly out of the remit of a care worker and so have not been included in this text. Of course, further, detailed training could be provided if required.

When dispensing medication in a care setting a system known as Monitored Dosage System (MDS) can aid with administration. It helps keep track of multiple medication administrations for individuals or for groups of individuals. It operates under a 7 or 28 day cycle and is generally only used for solid oral medication only. Other methods of administration are used for other forms of medication so extra care must be taken to ensure proper protocols are followed to avoid errors. Generally the MDS consists of rows and columns of compartments where each day's medication is put into compartments along a row according to the time they are due to be taken

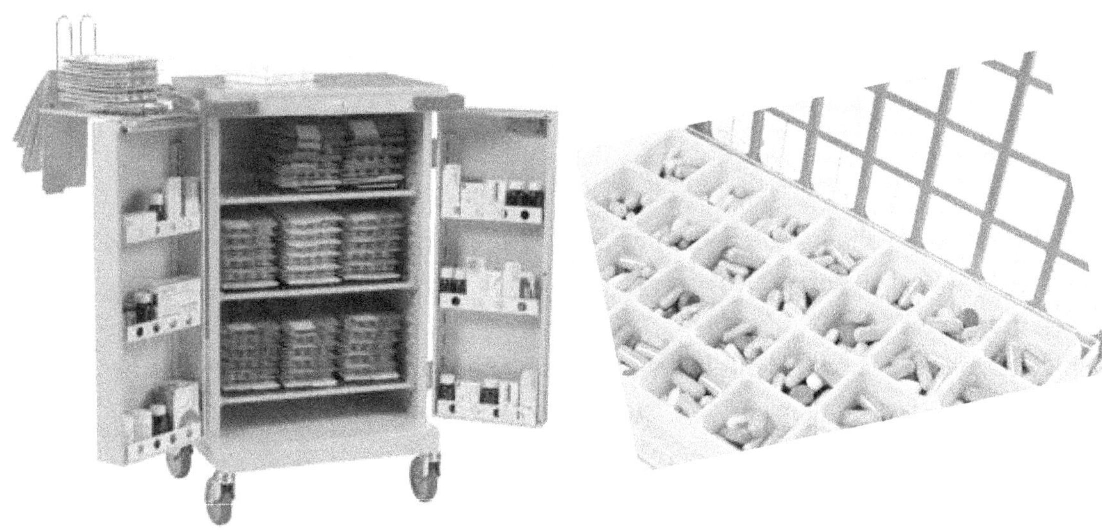

All medication also has an expiry date and this must be checked on a regular basis, it is normally 8 weeks once medication has been dispensed in MDS, this can lead to an increase in medication waste, particularly for PRN (or "as needed") medication and where medication is not given routinely at set times of the day.

Any tablets or capsules that cannot be identified and are similar to each other should not be placed together in a MDS.

All medication must be identifiable and the description labelled by the pharmacist.

If there are any irregularities in the labelling, the medication should not be administered

and a manager should be informed at once.

Before embarking on a programme of self-administration (with or without supervision) it is advisable to offer a teaching and advisory programme. This allows patients to:

- Gain a better understanding of their medicines
- Practice the administration of their medicines
- Identify with health care staff medication problems at an early stage
- Have greater independence and empowerment
- Improve trust and consequently their relationship with health care staff

It is impossible to completely eliminate the element of risk that accompanies any system of medicine administration but careful selection of the patient and setting up appropriate controls, the risks of self-administration can be minimised. The following tactics will also assist in delivering a robust self-administration regime:

- Appropriate assessment of the candidate's ability to act in a way that wont risk harming themselves or others.
- Good collaboration and effective communication with the multidisciplinary care team
- Clearly defined roles and responsibilities and well prepared procedures
- Valid consent gives patients responsibility for medicine administration.

All individuals should be encouraged to self-administer if possible

Compliance Checks

Once it is agreed that the individual may self-administer compliance check will need to be done in a particular way:

1. Give the individual the medication and record the quantity given on the MAR chart (each individual must still have a record of all prescribed medicines).
2. After four or five days calculate the number of tablets that should have been taken and how many should be left in the box then check the actual number of tablets with the individual.
3. Record this compliance check for each medicine on the MAR chart.
4. Where possible no one should ever secondary dispense (manually enter medication into MDS) because of the risk of error.
5. Dosette boxes, which are stored in in a locked trolley, should always be taken to the patient before dispensing rather than dispensing the pills of different patients into pots and carried to the patients on a tray. The potential for errors in this case is far too great.
6. **If it is apparent that the individual has not taken their medication correctly reassess their support needs (blister packs, for instance) or suspend the self-administration pending further review with their GP. *This system is not suitable for everyone.***

A PEG is a feeding tube which passes through the abdominal wall directly into the stomach, so that nutrition can be provided without swallowing, or in some cases to supplement ordinary food. The PEG tube can be connected to a 'giving set' to provide feeds continuously or a syringe can be used to receive feeds at intervals. Medical professionals may also prescribe certain medication be delivered using this method either in single doses or continuously through a feeding set.

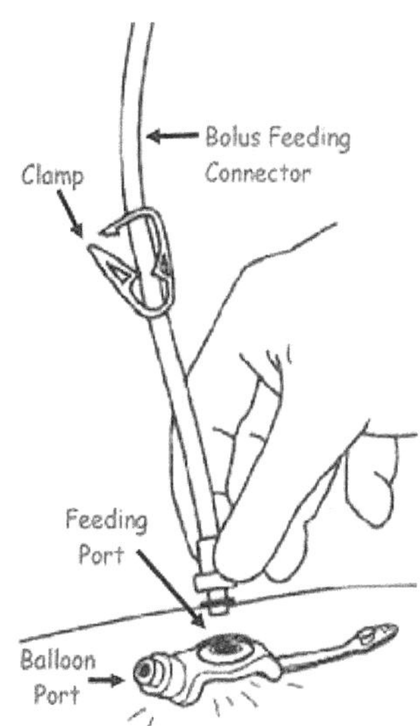

As this is quite a specialised area it is advisable to receive hands on training before admininstering medication in this way.

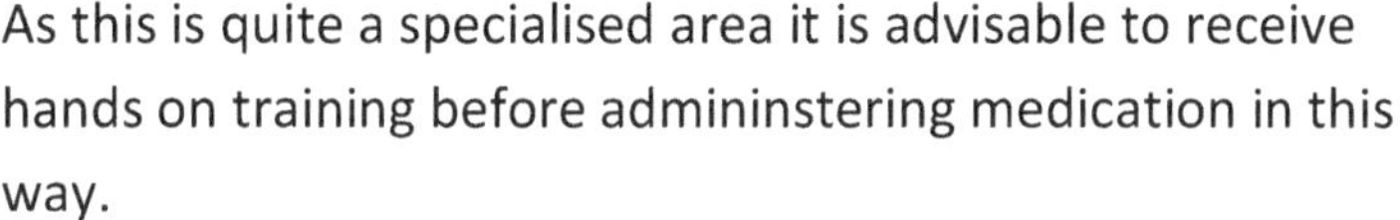

One of the most important things patients/carers need to be taught is caring for the feeding tube correctly. This includes flushing the tube with water immediately after any feed or medication has been administered via it. The most common cause of blocked tubes is leaving too long a time between feeding and flushing. Should a tube block, there are a variety of different tactics which may help unblock it including flushing with fizzy drinks, pineapple juice or sodium bicarbonate, whilst manipulating the tube between the fingers. There are also enzyme preparations which can be used in extreme cases. Inserting a sharp object down the tube to remove a blockage is discouraged.

(http://www.dietetics.co.uk)

Note: Crushing a tablet or opening a capsule makes its use unlicensed, therefore it is illegal to do so, if this needs to be done you must obtain the prescriber's authorisation in writing. An alternative formula should be found.

Common side effects

All medication has the potential to cause side effects, some of which can be extremely distressing and dangerous, even potentially fatal in the elderly or those with lowered immune systems. Accordingly it is important that the carer is aware of the potential for side effects and be prepared to assist as required.

The role of the carer is to administer the medication and observe if any side effects appear, and, if they do, report, record and seek medical advice as needed.
Any side effects must be reported to a manager or GP so that alternative medication or other solution may be found.

Some common side effects include:
- Drowsiness
- Being less alert
- Tiredness
- Difficulty concentrating
- Slurred or impaired speech
- Mood swings
- Tremors or shakes
- Slowed reaction times
- Decreased physical coordination
- Stiffness
- Swelling
- Vomiting
- Diarrhoea
- Headaches
- Rashes

This list of common side effects is not an exhaustive one and all side effects must be recorded on the relevant care plan or MAR in addition to informing a manager or GP.

A more serious reaction to medication can take place in the form of anaphylactic shock, for example. Situations such as these require professional medical attention and it is important to know how to react. The carer should:
1. Inform the manager and seek professional medical attention.
2. Observe the individual till help arrives (*they may need to administer CPR)*
3. Record all adverse reaction for future reference
4. If treatment is not possible in the home, take the patient to the hospital
5. Inform the GP and pharmacist if not done so
6. Inform medical staff of all the medication the person is taking including the medication believed to have caused the serious reaction

With the best will in the world errors do occur and the care industry is not exempt from these. They must, however, be dealt with swiftly and appropriately to prevent the situation from becoming worse, even causing a fatality.

Honesty is the best policy - Do not attempt to cover it up or lie!

When it is believed that someone may have taken a drugs overdose, whether intentionally or accidentally, help must be summoned immediately.

- Stay calm
- Ring 999
- Try to keep the person awake
- Do not walk them around
- Give the paramedics a list of the medication you believe they have taken and any other information you think may be relevant
- If they stop breathing start resuscitation

As soon after the incident as possible make a detailed record of the event and make sure that all relevant information is recorded in the care plan.

If the individual has indented to harm themselves, ongoing treatment may be required which may involve the support of

- Care manager and staff
- The GP
- A psychologist
- A psychiatrist
- Family and friends
- An advocate

By working as a team a service user will receive the correct treatment and support.

> **Hazardous Waste Regulations (2005)**
>
> This defines household and industrial waste and includes medicines that are no longer required. For example, care homes with nursing in England and Wales must use a clinical waste company to dispose of unwanted medicines. Care homes without nursing can return medicines to the supplying pharmacy for destruction.

Note: Medication is also recognised as a hazardous substance.

Disposal of Medication

Not all the medication that is prescribed will be used for a number of reasons including the fact that it has expired or is no longer being used due to a change in prescription. In these situations the waste medication must be disposed of in the correct manner. It must be disposed of as soon as possible and the care home will have *policies and procedures that clearly sets out guidelines to follow*.

Below is a list of some of the points to consider when disposing of medication safely:

- Liquid waste must be placed in a special bin, not poured down sinks or toilets.
- All transdermal patches must be folded in half render them ineffective.
- All clinical waste boxes should still be kept in a locked cupboard till they are removed by an authorised person.
- All medication that is no longer required must be logged in the return book.
- The disposal of controlled drugs must be monitored strictly to ensure that all medicines are accounted for. All details must be entered into the CD register and signed off by two authorised people.
- A pharmacist cannot collect waste from any care home that provides nursing care or a combination of nursing and personal care. In these cases all medicine must be taken out of their boxes (but not removed from their blister packs) and placed in the bin designed for waste. A clinical waste company will then collect all waste medication.
- A pharmacist can collect waste from a care home that does not provide nursing services and in these cases medication can be left in their containers and placed in the bin specifically for collection by the pharmacists.

When you are dealing with the disposal of sharps it is essential to be vigilant and pay attention. Lapses in concentration could result in a serious accident.

Needles and syringes must be placed in a specially provided "sharps box" after use. This will reduce the risk of stick injuries and cross contamination. In the event of a needle stick injury, however, the following steps should be taken:

- Encourage wound to bleed ideally by holding under a running tap.
- Wash the area well with soap and water
- Dry and cover
- Go immediately to the Emergency Department of your local hospital.
- **DO NOT SCRUB**
- **DO NOT SUCK**
- **DO NOT WASH WITH BLEACH**
- As soon after the incident as possible inform the Occupational Health Department.

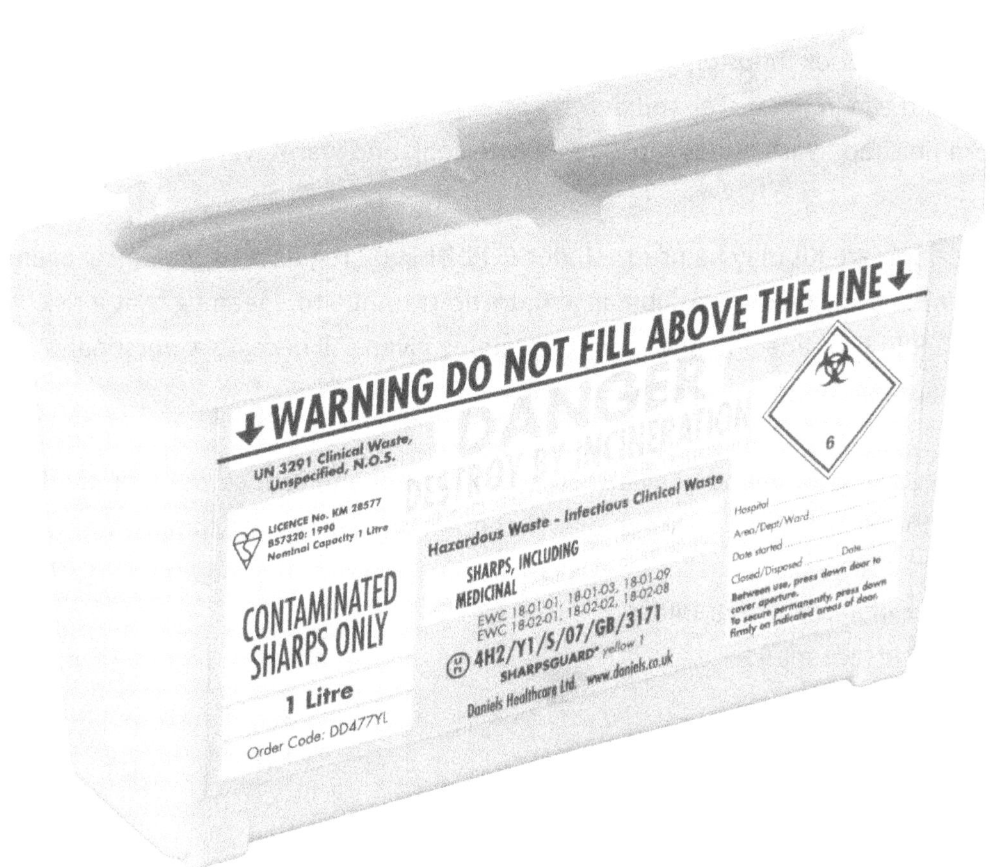

Disposal of Spills

Work areas should always be well maintained and kept hygienic. However accidents do occur and spillages can happen. When dealing with any hazardous substances it is important to use the correct equipment when dealing with the clean-up. This may involve gloves and aprons, masks and a spillage kit. The care home should also have put into place policies and procedures to deal with the clean-up of spills in order to protect their staff. These should be checked and understood before attempting to clean up a spill.

When dealing with spills of blood or other bodily fluids:
- Wear disposable gloves or rubber work gloves and, if there is risk of splashing, protective eye wear.
- Use disposable absorbent material, such as paper towels, to clean most of the spill. Place these in a plastic bag and put in the clinical waste bin.
- Clean the surface using soap and water to remove any remaining blood or body fluids.
- Wipe contaminated surfaces with a disinfectant solution. Mixing 1 part of household bleach to 50 parts of water makes a good solution. This type of bleach solution should be made freshly before use or it may lose its strength. For carpets or upholstery damaged by bleach, other household germicides or disinfectant agents can be used. Soak mops or cloths used for cleaning in a disinfectant for 20 minutes or wash these in hot water and detergent.
- When finished, wash hands thoroughly with soap and warm water.

Alternatively a Spillage Kit may be used. Under COSHH 2002 regulations biological agents such as present in body fluid are a substance hazardous to health, meaning that a risk assessment should be made and any required training given. All necessary personal protective equipment must be supplied.

The spillage kits are recommended as a method to control and reduce the risk of infection as required by the Health and Safety Act. It will contain two sealed kits comprising:

1 X 10g pack of absorbent granules

1 X disposable face mask

1 X disposable apron

1 X plastic scoop and scraper

1 X pair of disposable latex gloves

1 X non-alcoholic hand wipe

1 X disposable cleaning cloth

1 X 30ml viruscidal cleaning fluid.

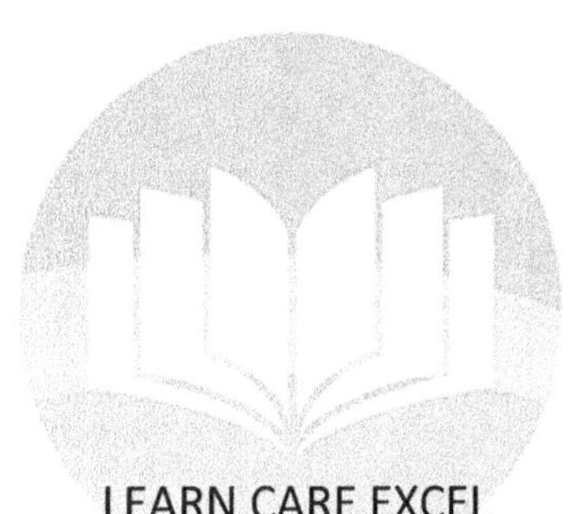

Matthews House
21 Thorley Park Road
Bishops Stortford
CM23 3NG

Tel: 07774 880880

info@learncareexcel.co.uk
www.learncareexcel.co.uk